Slow Cooker Meals

Super Tasty and affordable Snack &

Appetizers for beginners

Donna Conway

implied. readers acknowledge that the author is not engaging in the rendering of legal, financial, medical or professional advice. the content within this book has been derived from various sources. please consult a licensed professional before attempting any techniques outlined in this book.

by reading this document, the reader agrees that under no circumstances is the author responsible for any losses, direct or indirect, which are incurred as a result of the use of information contained within this document, including, but not limited to, — errors, omissions, or inaccuracies.

Table of Contents

Treacle Sponge with Honey

Preparation time: 15 minutes

Cooking time: 3 hours

Servings: 4 people

Ingredients:

- 1 cup unsalted butter

- 3 tbsp. honey

- 1 tbsp. white breadcrumbs (fresh)

- 1 cup of sugar

- 1 lemon zest

- 3 large chicken eggs

- 2 cup flour

- 2 tbsp. milk

- Clotted cream (to serve)

- Little brandy splash (optional)

Directions:

1. Grease your slow cooker dish heavily and preheat it. Mix the breadcrumbs with the honey in a medium bowl. Melt butter and beat it with lemon zest and sugar until fluffy and light. Sift in the flour slowly.

2. Add the milk and stir well. Spoon the mixture into the slow cooker dish. Cook for 3 hours on low mode. Serve with honey or clotted cream.

Nutrition:

Calories: 200

Fat: 10g

Carbs: 20g

Protein: 10g

Sticky Pecan Buns with Maple

Preparation time: 15 minutes

Cooking time: 5 hours

Servings: 12 rolls

Ingredients:

- 6 tbsp. milk (nonfat)

- 4 tbsp. maple syrup

- 1/2 tbsp. melted butter

- 1 tsp. vanilla extract

- Salt

- 2 tbsp. yeast

- 2 cup flour (whole wheat)

- Chopped pecans

- Ground cinnamon

Directions:

1. Coat the inside of your slow cooker using a non-stick cooking spray. For the dough, combine milk, vanilla butter, and maple syrup. Mix well.

2. Microwave the mixture until warm and add the yeast. Let sit for 15 minutes. Sift in the flour and mix until the dough is no stickier.

3. For the filling, mix the maple syrup and cinnamon. Roll out the dough and brush it with the maple filling. Roll up, then slice into 10-12 parts. Place the small rolls into the slow cooker.

4. For the caramel sauce, combine milk, butter, and syrup. Pour the sauce into the slow cooker. Cook for 2 hours on high or 5 hours on low. Serve.

Nutrition: Calories: 230, Fat: 5g, Carbs: 29g, Protein: 42g

Vegetarian Pot Pie

Preparation time: 15 minutes

Cooking time: 9 hours & 15 minutes

Servings: 4 people

Ingredients:

- 6 cups chopped vegetables (peas, potatoes, tomatoes, carrots, brussels sprouts)

- 1-2 cups diced mushrooms

- 2 onions

- 1/2 cup flour

- 4 cloves garlic

- 2 tbsp. garlic

- Thyme (fresh)

- Cornstarch

- 2 cups chicken broth

Directions:

1. Wash and chop vegetables or by frozen packed. Toss with flour to cover vegetables well.

2. Mix with the broth slowly, when well combined with flour. Preheat the slow cooker and place the vegetables into it.

3. Cook on low for 8-9 hours, or on high for 6-7 hours. Mix up cornstarch with the water and pour into the vegetable mix. Place it back in the slow cooker for 15 minutes. Serve hot with fresh vegetables.

Nutrition: Calories: 267, Fat: 7g, Carbs: 29g, Protein: 7g

Blueberry Porridge

Preparation time: 5 minutes

Cooking time: 5-6 hours

Servings: 4 people

Ingredients:

- 1 cup jumbo oats

- 4 cups of milk

- 1/2 cup dried fruits

- Brown sugar or honey

- Cinnamon

- Blueberries

Directions:

1. Heat the slow cooker before the start. Put the oats into the slow cooker dish, add some salt.

2. Pour over the milk, then place the dish into the slow cooker and cook on low for 7-8 hours (overnight). Stir the porridge in the morning.

3. For serving, ladle into the serving bowls and decorate with your favorite yogurt or syrup. Add blueberries.

Nutrition:

Calories: 210

Fat: 4g

Carbs: 5g

Protein: 8g

Cauliflower and Eggs Bowls

Preparation time: 15 minutes

Cooking time: 7 hours

Servings: 2 people

Ingredients:

- Cooking spray

- 4 eggs, whisked

- A pinch of salt and black pepper

- ¼ teaspoon thyme, dried

- ½ teaspoon turmeric powder

- 1 cup cauliflower florets

- ½ small yellow onion, chopped

- 3 oz. breakfast sausages, sliced

- ½ cup cheddar cheese, shredded

Directions:

1. Oiled your slow cooker with cooking spray and spread the cauliflower florets on the bottom of the pot. Add the eggs mixed with salt, pepper, and the other ingredients and toss. Put the lid on, cook on low for 7 hours, divide between plates, and serve for breakfast.

Nutrition:

Calories: 261

Fat: 6g

Carbs: 22g

Protein: 6g

Milk Oatmeal

Preparation time: 10 minutes

Cooking time: 2 hours

Servings: 4 people

Ingredients:

- 2 cups oatmeal

- 1 cup of water

- 1 cup milk

- 1 tablespoon liquid honey

- 1 teaspoon vanilla extract

- 1 tablespoon coconut oil

- ¼ teaspoon ground cinnamon

Directions:

1. Put all ingredients except liquid honey in the slow cooker and mix. Cook the meal on high for hours.

2. Then stir the cooked oatmeal and transfer to the serving bowls. Top the meal with a small amount of liquid honey.

Nutrition:

Calories: 234

Protein: 7.4g

Carbs: 35.3g

Fat: 7.3g

Asparagus Egg Casserole

Preparation time: 15 minutes

Cooking time: 2 hours & 30 minutes

Servings: 4 people

Ingredients:

- 7 eggs, beaten

- 4 oz asparagus, chopped, boiled

- 1 oz Parmesan, grated

- 1 teaspoon sesame oil

- 1 teaspoon dried dill

Directions:

1. Pour the sesame oil into the slow cooker. Then mix dried dill with parmesan, asparagus, and eggs. Pour the egg batter into your slow cooker and close the lid.

Cook the casserole on high for 2 hours and 30 minutes. Serve.

Nutrition:

Calories: 149

Protein: 12.6g

Carbs: 2.1g

Fat: 10.3g

Vanilla Maple Oats

Preparation time: 15 minutes

Cooking time: 8 hours

Servings: 4 people

Ingredients:

- 1 cup steel-cut oats

- 2 tsp vanilla extract

- 2 cups vanilla almond milk

- 2 tbsp maple syrup

- 2 tsp cinnamon powder

- 2 cups of water

- 2 tsp flaxseed

- Cooking spray

- 2 tbsp blackberries

Directions:

1. Coat the base of your slow cooker with cooking spray. Stir in oats, almond milk, vanilla extract, cinnamon, maple syrup, flaxseeds, and water.

2. Put the cooker's lid on and set the cooking time to 8 hours on low. Stir well and serve with blackberries on top. Devour.

Nutrition:

Calories: 200

Fat: 3g

Carbs: 9g

Protein: 3g

Raspberry Oatmeal

Preparation time: 15 minutes

Cooking time: 8 hours

Servings: 4 people

Ingredients:

- 2 cups of water

- 1 tablespoon coconut oil

- 1 cup steel-cut oats

- 1 tablespoon sugar

- 1 cup milk

- ½ teaspoon vanilla extract

- 1 cup raspberries

- 4 tablespoons walnuts, chopped

Directions:

1. In your slow cooker, mix oil with water, oats, sugar, milk, vanilla, and raspberries, cover, and cook on low for 8 hours. Stir oatmeal, divide into bowls, sprinkle walnuts on top, and serve for breakfast.

Nutrition:

Calories: 200

Fat: 10g

Carbs: 20g

Protein: 4g

Pork and Eggplant Casserole

Preparation time: 15 minutes

Cooking time: 6 hours

Servings: 2 people

Ingredients:

- 1 red onion, chopped

- 1 eggplant, cubed

- ½ pound pork stew meat, ground

- 3 eggs, whisked

- ½ teaspoon chili powder

- ½ teaspoon garam masala

- 1 tablespoon sweet paprika

- 1 teaspoon olive oil

Directions:

1. Mix the eggs with the meat, onion, eggplant, and the other ingredients in the bowl except for the oil. Grease your slow cooker with oil, add the pork and eggplant mix, spread into the pot, cook on low for 6 hours. Divide the mixture between plates and serve for breakfast.

Nutrition:

Calories: 261

Fat: 7g

Carbs: 16g

Protein: 7g

Baby Spinach Rice Mix

Preparation time: 15 minutes

Cooking time: 6 hours

Servings: 4 people

Ingredients:

- ¼ cup mozzarella, shredded

- ½ cup baby spinach

- ½ cup wild rice

- 1 and ½ cups chicken stock

- ½ teaspoon turmeric powder

- ½ teaspoon oregano, dried

- A pinch of salt and black pepper

- 3 scallions, minced

- ¾ cup goat cheese, crumbled

Directions:

1. In your slow cooker, mix the rice with the stock, turmeric, and the other ingredients, toss, cook on low for 6 hours. Divide the mix into bowls and serve for breakfast.

Nutrition:

Calories: 165

Fat: 1.2g

Carbs: 32.6g

Protein: 7.6g

Baby Carrots in Syrup

Preparation time: 15 minutes

Cooking time: 7 hours

Servings: 4 people

Ingredients:

- 3 cups baby carrots

- 1 cup apple juice

- 2 tablespoons brown sugar

- 1 teaspoon vanilla extract

Directions:

1. Mix apple juice, brown sugar, and vanilla extract. Pour the liquid into the slow cooker. Add baby carrots and close the lid. Cook the meal on low for 7 hours.

Nutrition:

Calories: 81,

Protein: 0g,

Carbs: 18.8g,

Fat: 0.1g

Green Muffins

Preparation time: 15 minutes

Cooking time: 2 hours & 30 minutes

Servings: 8 muffins

Ingredients:

- 1 cup spinach, washed

- 5 tbsp butter

- 1 cup flour

- 1 tsp salt

- ½ tsp baking soda

- 1 tbsp lemon juice

- 1 tbsp sugar

- 3 eggs

-

Directions:

1. Add the spinach leaves to a blender jug and blend until smooth. Whisk the eggs in a bowl and add the spinach mixture.

2. Stir in baking soda, salt, sugar, flour, and lemon juice. Mix well to form a smooth spinach batter. Divide the dough into a muffin tray lined with muffin cups.

3. Place this muffin tray in the slow cooker. Put the cooker's lid on and set the cooking time to 2 hours 30 minutes on high. Serve.

Nutrition:

Calories: 172

Fat: 6.1g

Carbs: 9.23g

Protein: 20g

Scallions and Bacon Omelet

Preparation time: 15 minutes

Cooking time: 2 hours

Servings: 4 people

Ingredients:

- 5 eggs, beaten

- 2 oz bacon, chopped, cooked

- 1 oz scallions, chopped

- 1 teaspoon olive oil

- ½ teaspoon ground black pepper

- ¼ teaspoon cayenne pepper

Directions:

1. Brush the slow cooker bowl bottom with olive oil. After this, mix eggs with bacon, scallions, ground black pepper, and cayenne pepper in the bowl. Pour the liquid into your slow cooker and close the lid. Cook the meal on high for 2 hours. Serve.

Nutrition:

Calories: 169

Protein: 12.3g

Carbs: 1.4g

Fat: 12.6g

Cowboy Breakfast Casserole

Preparation time: 15 minutes

Cooking time: 3 hours

Servings: 4 people

Ingredients:

- 1-pound ground beef

- 5 eggs, beaten

- 1 cup grass-fed Monterey Jack cheese, shredded

- Salt and pepper to taste

- 1 avocado, peeled and diced

- A handful of cilantros, chopped

- A dash of hot sauce

Directions:

1. In a skillet over medium flame, sauté the beef for three minutes until slightly golden. Pour into the slow cooker and pour in eggs.

2. Sprinkle with cheese on top and season with salt and pepper to taste. Close the lid and cook on high for hours or on low for 6 hours. Serve with avocado, cilantro, and hot sauce.

Nutrition:

Calories: 439

Carbs: 4.5g

Protein: 32.7g

Fat: 31.9g

Maple Banana Oatmeal

Preparation time: 15 minutes

Cooking time: 6 hours

Servings: 2 people

Ingredients:

- 1/2 cup old fashioned oats

- 1 banana, mashed

- ½ teaspoon cinnamon powder

- 2 tablespoons maple syrup

- 2 cups almond milk

- Cooking spray

Directions:

1. Grease your slow cooker with the cooking spray, add the oats, banana, and the other ingredients, stir, cook

on low for 6 hours. Divide into bowls and serve for breakfast.

Nutrition:

Calories: 815

Fat: 60.3g

Carbs: 67g

Protein: 11.1g

Potato Muffins

Preparation time: 15 minutes

Cooking time: 2 hours

Servings: 4 people

Ingredients:

- 4 teaspoons flax meal

- 1 bell pepper, diced

- 1 cup potato, cooked, mashed

- 2 eggs, beaten

- 1 teaspoon ground paprika

- 2 oz Mozzarella, shredded

Directions:

1. Mix flax meal with potato and eggs. Then add ground paprika and bell pepper. Stir the mixture with the help of the spoon until homogenous.

2. Transfer the potato mixture to the muffin molds. Top the muffins with mozzarella and transfer them to the slow cooker. Close the lid and cook the muffins on high for 2 hours. Serve.

Nutrition:

Calories: 107

Protein: 8g

Carbs: 7.2g

Fat: 5.7g

Eggs and Sweet Potato Mix

Preparation time: 15 minutes

Cooking time: 6 hours

Servings: 2 people

Ingredients:

- ½ red onion, chopped

- ½ green bell pepper, chopped

- 2 sweet potatoes, peeled and grated

- ½ red bell pepper, chopped

- 1 garlic clove, minced

- ½ teaspoon olive oil

- 4 eggs, whisked

- 1 tablespoon chives, chopped

- A pinch of red pepper, crushed

- A pinch of salt and black pepper

Directions:

1. Mix the eggs with the onion, bell peppers, and the other ingredients in a bowl except for the oil.

2. Grease your slow cooker with the oil, add the eggs and potato mix, spread, cook on low within 6 hours. Divide everything between plates and serve.

Nutrition:

Calories: 261

Fat: 6g

Carbs: 16g

Protein: 4g

Veggie Hash Brown Mix

Preparation time: 15 minutes

Cooking time: 6 hours & 5 minutes

Servings: 2 people

Ingredients:

- 1 tablespoon olive oil

- ½ cup white mushrooms, chopped

- ½ yellow onion, chopped

- ¼ teaspoon garlic powder

- ¼ teaspoon onion powder

- ¼ cup sour cream

- 10 oz. hash browns

- ¼ cup cheddar cheese, shredded

- Salt and black pepper to the taste

- ½ tablespoon parsley, chopped

Directions:

1. Heat-up a pan with the oil over medium heat, add the onion and mushrooms, stir and cook for 5 minutes.

2. Transfer this to the slow cooker, add hash browns and the other ingredients, toss, cook on low within 6 hours. Divide between plates and for breakfast.

Nutrition:

Calories: 571

Fat: 35.6g

Carbs: 54.9g

Protein: 9.7g

Coconut Cranberry Quinoa

Preparation time: 5 minutes

Cooking time: 2 hours

Servings: 4 people

Ingredients:

- 3 cups of coconut water

- 1 cup quinoa, uncooked and rinsed

- 3 teaspoons honey

- ¼ cup cranberries

- ½ cup coconut flakes

Directions:

1. Place all ingredients in the slow cooker. Add a dash of vanilla or cinnamon if desired. Give a good stir. Cook on low within 2 hours. Serve.

Nutrition:

Calories: 246

Carbs: 42g

Protein: 8g

Fat: 5g

Scrambled Eggs in Ramekins

Preparation time: 5 minutes

Cooking time: 4 hours

Servings: 2 people

Ingredients:

- 2 eggs, beaten

- ¼ cup milk

- Salt and pepper

- ¼ cup cheddar cheese, grated

- ½ cup of salsa

Directions:

1. Mix the eggs and milk in a mixing bowl. Season with salt and pepper to taste. Place egg mixture in two ramekins. Sprinkle with cheddar cheese on top.

2. Put the ramekins in the slow cooker, then pour water around it. Cook on low within 4 hours. Serve with salsa.

Nutrition:

Calories: 243

Carbs: 9.3g

Protein: 15.3g

Fat: 164g

Enchilada Breakfast Casserole

Preparation time: 5 minutes

Cooking time: 10 hours

Servings: 4 people

Ingredients:

- 6 eggs, beaten

- 1-pound ground beef

- 2 cans enchilada sauce

- 1 can condensed cream of onion soup

- 3 cups sharp cheddar cheese, grated

Directions:

1. Beat the eggs, then season with salt plus pepper in a mixing bowl. Set aside. In a skillet, brown the beef for at least 5 minutes.

2. Pour the beef into the slow cooker and stir in the enchilada sauce and cream of onion soup. Stir in the eggs and place cheese on top. Cook on low within 10 hours. Serve.

Nutrition:

Calories: 320

Carbs: 9.4g

Protein: 24.6g

Fat: 20.1g

White Chocolate Oatmeal

Preparation time: 5 minutes

Cooking time: 4 hours

Servings: 4 people

Ingredients:

- 1 tablespoon white chocolate chips

- 1 cup of water

- ½ cup oatmeal

- 1 tablespoon brown sugar

- 1 teaspoon cinnamon

Directions:

1. Stir in all fixing in the slow cooker. Cook on low within 4 hours. Top with your favorite topping.

Nutrition: Calories: 31, Carbs: 5.4g, Protein: 0.5g, Fat: 0.9g

Bacon-Wrapped Hotdogs

Preparation time: 15 minutes

Cooking time: 8 hours

Servings: 4 people

Ingredients:

- 8 small hotdogs

- 8 bacon

- ½ cup brown sugar

- 4 tablespoons water

- Salt and pepper to taste

Directions:

1. Wrap the individual hotdogs with bacon strips. Secure with a toothpick, then place inside the slow cooker.

2. Mix the sugar, water, salt, and pepper in a small mixing bowl. Pour over the hotdogs. Cook on low within 8 hours. Serve.

Nutrition:

Calories: 120

Carbs: 11.8g

Protein: 3.1g

Fat: 6.9g

Apple Granola Crumble

Preparation time: 15 minutes

Cooking time: 3 hours

Servings: 4 people

Ingredients:

- 2 Granny Smith apples, cored and sliced

- 1 cup granola cereal

- 1/8 cup maple syrup

- ¼ cup apple juice

- 1 teaspoon cinnamon

Directions:

1. Place all ingredients in the slow cooker. Give a good stir. Cook on low within 3 hours. Once cooked, serve with a tablespoon of butter.

Nutrition: Calories: 369,

Carbs: 56g,

Protein: 5g,

Fat:15g

Banana and Coconut Milk Steel-Cut Oats

Preparation time: 15 minutes

Cooking time: 3 hours

Servings: 4 people

Ingredients:

- 2 medium ripe bananas, sliced

- 2 cans coconut milk, unsweetened

- 1 cup steel-cut oats

- 2 tablespoons brown sugar

- ½ teaspoon cinnamon

Directions:

1. Place all ingredients in the slow cooker. Add a dash of salt if needed. Give a good stir. Cook on low within 3

hours. Once cooked, serve with a tablespoon of melted butter.

Nutrition:

Calories:101

Carbs: 15.3g

Protein: 2.6g

Fat: 5.9g

Spinach and Mozzarella Frittata

Preparation time: 10 minutes

Cooking time: 4 hours

Servings: 4 people

Ingredients:

- 6 eggs, beaten
- 2 tablespoons milk
- 1 cup baby spinach
- 1 cup mozzarella cheese
- 1 Roma tomatoes, diced

Directions:

1. Mix the eggs and milk in a mixing bowl. Season with salt and pepper to taste. Put the egg batter into the slow cooker and add the baby spinach, cheese, and tomatoes. Cook on low within 4 hours.

Nutrition:

Calories: 139,

Carbs: 4g,

Protein: 12g,

Fat: 8g

Quinoa Energy Bars

Preparation time: 15 minutes

Cooking time: 8 hours

Servings: 4 people

Ingredients:

- 2 cups quinoa flakes, rinsed
- ½ cup nuts of your choice
- ½ cup dried fruits of your choice
- ¼ cup butter, melted
- 1/3 cup maple syrup

Directions:

1. In a mixing bowl, combine all ingredients. Compress the fixing in a parchment-lined slow cooker. Cook on low within 8 hours.

Nutrition:

Calories: 306,

Carbs: 39.9g,

Protein: 7.3g,

Fat: 13.9g

Overnight Apple Oatmeal

Preparation time: 15 minutes

Cooking time: 8 hours

Servings: 4 people

Ingredients:

- 4 apples, peeled and diced

- ¾ cup brown sugar

- 2 cups old-fashioned oats

- 4 cups evaporated milk

- 1 tablespoon cinnamon

Directions:

1. Stir in all fixing in the slow cooker. Cook on low within 8 hours. Add in butter if desired.

Nutrition: Calories: 521, Carbs: 109.5g, Protein: 16.4g

Fat: 11.6

Apple Walnut Strata

Preparation time: 15 minutes

Cooking time: 2 hours

Servings: 4 people

Ingredients:

- ¼ cup light cream

- ¼ cup of orange juice

- 3 eggs, beaten

- 3 tablespoons sugar

- ½ teaspoon cinnamon

- 1 teaspoon vanilla

- 4 cups cubed French bread

- 1 cup granola

- ½ cup chopped toasted walnuts

- 2 Granny Smith apples, peeled and cubed

Directions:

1. Oiled 3 or 4-quart slow cooker using a nonstick cooking spray. In a medium bowl, combine cream, orange juice, eggs, sugar, cinnamon, and vanilla and blend well with a whisk. Set aside.

2. Place the bread in the prepared slow cooker's bottom and sprinkle it with the granola, walnuts, and apples—repeat layers. Pour egg mixture overall. Cover and cook on high within 1½ to 2 hours or until just set. Serve.

Nutrition:

Calories: 357.67

Fat: 16.56g

Protein: 11.97 g

Carbs: 0g

Nutty Oatmeal

Preparation time: 15 minutes

Cooking time: 9 hours & 9 minutes

Servings: 4 people

Slow cooker size: 3 1/2-quart

Ingredients:

- 1½ cups steel-cut oatmeal
- 2 tablespoons butter
- 1 cup chopped walnuts
- 6 cups of water
- ½ cup brown sugar
- 1 teaspoon salt
- 1 teaspoon cinnamon
- 1 teaspoon nutmeg

Directions:

1. Put the oatmeal in a large skillet over medium-high heat. Toast, continually stirring, for 8–9 minutes or until oatmeal is fragrant and begins to brown around the edges. Remove to 3½-quart slow cooker.

2. Dissolve butter and add chopped walnuts in the same pan. Toast over medium heat, continually stirring, until nuts are toasted.

3. Combine with all remaining ingredients except spices in 3– the 4-quart slow cooker. Cover and cook on low for 7–9 hours, until oatmeal is tender.

4. Stir in spices, cover, and let stand for 10 minutes. Serve topped with a bit of butter, maple syrup, brown sugar, and more chopped nuts.

Nutrition: Calories: 388, Carbs: 32g, Fat: 26g, Protein: 13g

Bacon and Waffle Strata

Preparation time: 15 minutes

Cooking time: 5 hours

Servings: 4 people

Ingredients:

- 4 slices bacon

- 5 frozen waffles, toasted

- 1 cup shredded Colby cheese

- ¼ cup chopped green onions

- 1 (5-ounce) can evaporate milk

- ½ package cream cheese softened

- 4 eggs

- ½ teaspoon dry mustard

Directions:

1. Cook bacon until crisp in your large skillet. Drain on paper towels, crumble, and set aside. Cut toasted

waffles into cubes. Layer bacon and waffle cubes with cheese and green onions in a 3½-quart slow cooker.

2. Drain skillet, discarding bacon fat; do not wipe out. Put the milk plus cream cheese in skillet; cook over low heat, stirring frequently.

3. Remove, then beat in eggs, one at a time, until smooth. Stir in dry mustard, then pour into a slow cooker. Cover and cook on low within 4–5 hours, until eggs are set. Serve with warmed maple syrup, if desired.

Nutrition: Calories: 382, Carbs: 25g, Fat: 22g, Protein: 21g

Honey Apple Bread Pudding

Preparation time: 15 minutes

Cooking time: 4 hours & 35 minutes

Servings: 4 people

Ingredients:

- 2 apples, chopped
- ¼ cup apple juice
- cup brown sugar
- ¼ cup honey
- 2 tablespoons butter, melted
- 4 eggs, beaten
- cup whole milk
- 1 teaspoon vanilla
- ½ teaspoon cinnamon
- 8 slices raisin swirl bread
- ½ cup raisin

Directions:

1. In a medium saucepan, combine apples with apple juice. Bring to a simmer; simmer for 5 minutes, stirring frequently. Remove, then set aside within 10 minutes. Drain apples, reserving juice.

2. Mix brown sugar, honey, and butter in a small bowl; set aside. In a large bowl, combine reserved apple juice, eggs, milk, vanilla, and cinnamon; beat well and set aside.

3. Cut bread slices into cubes. In the slow cooker, layer the bread cubes, raisins, apples, and the brown sugar mixture. Repeat layers. Pour egg mixture overall.

4. Cover and cook on high within 3 to 4 hours and 30 minutes, until pudding is set. Let cool within 30 minutes, then serve.

Nutrition:

Calories: 312, Carbs: 41g, Fat: 15g, Protein: 7g

Sausage Rolls

Preparation time: 15 minutes

Cooking time: 9 hours & 6 minutes

Servings: 4 people

Ingredients:

- ¾ cup soft bread crumbs
- 1 egg, beaten
- ¼ cup brown sugar
- ¼ cup applesauce
- ½ teaspoon salt
- 1 teaspoon pepper
- ½ teaspoon dried marjoram leaves
- 1½-pounds mild bulk pork sausage
- 2 tablespoons butter
- ¼ cup honey
- ¼ cup chicken broth

Directions:

1. In a large bowl, combine crumbs, egg, brown sugar, applesauce, salt, pepper, and marjoram. Mix well. Stir in sausage.

2. Shape into rolls 3" × 1". Dissolve the butter over medium heat in a large skillet. Add sausage rolls, about 8 at a time, and cook until browned on all sides, about 5–6 minutes.

3. As rolls cook, drain on paper towels, then place into the 3-quart slow cooker. In a small bowl, combine honey and chicken broth and mix well. Pour over sausage rolls in a slow cooker.

4. Cook on low within 8–9 hours or until sausage rolls are thoroughly cooked, to 165°F on a meat thermometer. Remove from slow cooker with a slotted spoon to serve.

Nutrition: Calories: 102, Carbs: 7g, Fat: 0g, Protein: 7g

Breakfast Pitas

Preparation time: 15 minutes

Cooking time: 7-8 hours & 5 minutes

Servings: 4 people

Ingredients:

- 2 tablespoons butter

- 1 onion, chopped

- 2 cloves garlic, chopped

- 8 eggs, beaten

- ½ teaspoon salt

- 1 teaspoon pepper

- ½ cup of salsa

- 1 cup shredded pepper jack cheese

- 4 pita bread

- 2 tablespoons chopped parsley

Directions:

1. Oiled 2-quart slow cooker with nonstick cooking spray. In a small skillet, melt butter over medium heat. Put the onion plus garlic; cook and stir until tender, about 5 minutes. Remove from heat.

2. Mix eggs, salt, and pepper and beat well in a large bowl. Stir in onion mixture, salsa, and cheese. Pour into the slow cooker. Cover and cook on low within 7–8 hours.

3. In the morning, stir the mixture in a slow cooker. Split pita bread and fill with egg mixture; top with parsley and serve immediately.

Nutrition:

Calories: 200

Carbs: 14g

Fat: 1g

Protein: 6g

Oregano Salsa

Preparation time: 10 minutes

Cooking time: 7 hours

Servings: 4 people

Ingredients:

- 3 cups eggplant, cubed

- 4 garlic cloves, minced

- 6 oz. green olives, pitted and sliced

- 1 and ½ cups tomatoes, chopped

- 2 teaspoons balsamic vinegar

- 1 tablespoon oregano, chopped

- Black pepper to the taste

Directions:

1. In your slow cooker, mix tomatoes with eggplant, green olives, garlic, vinegar, oregano, and pepper, toss, cover, cook on low for 7 hours, divide into small bowls and serve as an appetizer.

Nutrition:

Calories: 78

Fat: 3.6g

Carbs: 11.2g

Protein: 2g

Smoked Paprika Cauliflower Spread

Preparation time: 10 minutes

Cooking time: 7 hours

Servings: 4 people

Ingredients:

- 2 cups cauliflower florets

- 1 cup of coconut milk

- 1/3 cup cashews, chopped

- 2 and ½ cups of water

- 1 cup turnips, chopped

- 1 teaspoon garlic powder

- ¼ teaspoon smoked paprika

- ¼ teaspoon mustard powder

Directions:

1. In your slow cooker, mix cauliflower with cashews, turnips, and water, stir, cover, cook on low for 7 hours, drain, transfer to a blender, add milk, garlic powder, paprika, and mustard powder, blend well, and serve.

Nutrition:

Calories: 228

Fat: 19.7g

Carbs: 12.4g

Protein: 4.6g

French Style Salad

Preparation time: 10 minutes

Cooking time: 9 hours

Servings: 4 people

Ingredients:

- 6 oz. canned tomato paste, no-salt-added

- 2 tomatoes, cut into medium wedges

- 2 yellow onions, chopped

- 1 eggplant, sliced

- 4 zucchinis, sliced

- 2 green bell peppers, cut into medium strips

- 2 garlic cloves, minced

- 2 tablespoons parsley, chopped

- 3 tablespoons olive oil

- 1 teaspoon oregano, dried

- 1 tablespoon basil, chopped

- A pinch of black pepper

Directions:

1. In your slow cooker, mix oil with onions, eggplant, zucchinis, garlic, bell peppers, tomato paste, tomatoes, basil, oregano, and pepper, cover, and cook on low for 9 hours. Add parsley, toss, divide into small bowls and serve warm as an appetizer.

Nutrition:

Calories: 161

Fat: 7.8g

Carbs: 22.8g

Protein: 4.9g

Stevia and Bulgur Salad

Preparation time: 10 minutes

Cooking time: 12 hours

Servings: 4 people

Ingredients:

- 2 cups white mushrooms, sliced

- 14 oz. canned kidney beans, no-salt-added, drained

- 14 oz. canned pinto beans, no-salt-added, drained

- 2 cups yellow onion, chopped

- 1 cup low sodium veggie stock

- 1 cup strong coffee

- ¾ cup bulgur, soaked and drained

- ½ cup red bell pepper, chopped

- 2 garlic cloves, minced

- 2 tablespoons stevia

- 2 tablespoons chili powder

- 1 tablespoon cocoa powder

- 1 teaspoon oregano, dried

- 2 teaspoons cumin, ground

- Black pepper to the taste

Directions:

1. In your slow cooker, mix mushrooms with bulgur, onion, bell pepper, stock, garlic, coffee, kidney and pinto beans, stevia, chili powder, cocoa, oregano, cumin, and pepper, stir gently, cover, and cook on low for 12 hours. Divide the mix into small bowls and serve cold as an appetizer.

Nutrition:

Calories: 837

Fat: 4.2g

Carbs: 162g

Protein: 49.9g

Parmesan Stuffed Mushrooms

Preparation time: 10 minutes

Cooking time: 5 hours

Servings: 4 people

Ingredients:

- 20 mushrooms, stems removed

- 2 cups basil, chopped

- 1 cup tomato sauce, no-salt-added

- 2 tablespoons parsley, chopped

- ¼ cup low-fat parmesan, grated

- 1 and ½ cups whole wheat breadcrumbs

- 1 tablespoon garlic, minced

- ¼ cup low-fat butter, melted

- 2 teaspoons lemon juice

- 1 tablespoon olive oil

Directions:

1. In a bowl, mix butter with breadcrumbs and parsley, stir well, and leave aside. In your blender, mix basil with oil, parmesan, garlic, and lemon juice and pulse well.

2. Stuff mushrooms with this mix, pour the tomato sauce on top, sprinkle breadcrumbs mix at the end, and cook in the slow cooker on low for 5 hours. Arrange mushrooms on a platter and serve.

Nutrition:

Calories: 51

Fat: 1.1g

Carbs: 9g

Protein: 2.2g

Garlic and Tomato Appetizer

Preparation time: 10 minutes

Cooking time: 2 hours

Servings: 4 people

Ingredients:

- 2 teaspoons olive oil

- 8 tomatoes, chopped

- 1 garlic clove, minced

- ¼ cup basil, chopped

- 4 Italian whole wheat bread slices, toasted

- 3 tablespoons low-sodium veggie stock

- Black pepper to the taste

Directions:

1. In your slow cooker, mix tomatoes with basil, garlic, oil, veggie stock, and black pepper, stir, cover, cook on high within 2 hours and then leave aside to cool down. Divide this mix on the toasted bread and serve as an appetizer.

Nutrition:

Calories: 158

Fat: 4.1g

Carbs: 26.3g

Protein: 5.9g

Tahini Dip

Preparation time: 10 minutes

Cooking time: 3 hours

Servings: 4 people

Ingredients:

- ½ pound cauliflower florets

- 1 teaspoon avocado oil

- 1 tablespoon ginger, grated

- 1 cup coconut cream

- 3 garlic cloves, minced

- Black pepper to the taste

- 1 tablespoon basil, chopped

- 1 tablespoon tahini paste

- 1 tablespoon lime juice

Directions:

1. In your slow cooker, combine the cauliflower with the oil, ginger, and the other ingredients, cook on low within 3 hours. Transfer to your blender, pulse well, divide into bowls and serve.

Nutrition:

Calories: 217

Fat: 18.1g

Carbs: 13.3g

Protein: 3.7g

Lime Juice Snack

Preparation time: 10 minutes

Cooking time: 2 hours

Servings: 4 people

Ingredients:

- 1 pineapple, peeled and cut into medium sticks
- 2 tablespoons stevia
- 1 tablespoon olive oil
- 1 tablespoon lime juice
- 1 tablespoon lime zest, grated
- 1 teaspoon cinnamon powder
- ¼ teaspoon cloves, ground

Directions:

1. In a bowl, mix lime juice with stevia, oil, cinnamon, and cloves and whisk well. Add the pineapple sticks to your slow cooker, add lime mix, toss, cover, and cook on high for 2 hours. Serve the pineapple sticks as a snack with lime zest sprinkled on top.

Nutrition:

Calories: 26

Fat: 1.8g

Carbs: 6.1g

Protein: 0.1g

Cumin Hummus

Preparation time: 10 minutes

Cooking time: 5 hours

Servings: 4 people

Ingredients:

- 1 cup chickpeas, soaked overnight and drained
- 2 garlic cloves
- ¾ cup green onions, chopped
- 1 tablespoon olive oil
- 2 tablespoons sherry vinegar
- 3 cups of water
- 1 teaspoon cumin, ground

Directions:

1. Put the water in your slow cooker, add chickpeas and garlic, cover, and cook on low for 5 hours. Drain chickpeas, transfer them to your blender, add ½ cup of the cooking liquid, green onions, vinegar, oil,

cilantro, and cumin, blend well, divide into bowls and serve.

Nutrition:

Calories: 150

Fat: 4.5g

Carbs: 22.3g

Protein: 6.8g

Peppercorns Asparagus

Preparation time: 10 minutes

Cooking time: 2 hours

Servings: 4 people

Ingredients:

- 3 cups asparagus spears, halved

- 3 garlic cloves, sliced

- 1 tablespoon dill

- ¼ cup white wine vinegar

- ¼ cup apple cider vinegar

- 2 cloves

- 1 cup of water

- ¼ teaspoon red pepper flakes

- 8 black peppercorns

- 1 teaspoon coriander seeds

Directions:

1. In your slow cooker, mix the asparagus with the cider vinegar, white vinegar, dill, cloves, water, garlic, pepper flakes, peppercorns, and coriander, cover, and cook on high for 2 hours. Drain asparagus, transfer it to bowls, and serve as a snack.

Nutrition:

Calories: 20

Fat: 0.1g

Carbs: 3.6g

Protein: 1.7g

Light Shrimp Salad

Preparation time: 10 minutes

Cooking time: 5 hours and 30 minutes

Servings: 4 people

Ingredients:

- 1 cup tomato, chopped
- ¼ pound shrimp, peeled, deveined, and chopped
- 1 cup canned black beans, no-salt-added, drained and rinsed
- 1 cup cucumber, chopped
- 2 teaspoons cumin, ground
- 2 tablespoons olive oil
- ½ cup red onion, chopped
- Zest and juice of 2 limes
- Zest and juice of 2 lemons
- 2 tablespoons garlic, minced
- ¼ cup cilantro, chopped

Directions:

1. In a bowl, mix lime juice and lemon juice with shrimp and toss. Grease the slow cooker with the oil, add black beans, tomato, onion, garlic, and cumin, cover, and cook on low within 5 hours.

2. Add shrimp, cover, cook on low for 30 minutes, more, transfer everything to a bowl, add cucumber and cilantro, toss, leave aside to cool down, divide between small bowls and serve as an appetizer.

Nutrition:

Calories: 153

Fat: 4.4g

Carbs: 21.4g

Protein: 9.3g

Mushroom Salsa with Pumpkin Seeds

Preparation time: 10 minutes

Cooking time: 3 hours

Servings: 4 people

Ingredients:

- 1-pound white mushrooms, sliced

- 1 cup cherry tomatoes, halved

- 1 cup black olives, pitted and sliced

- 1 tablespoon olive oil

- Juice of 1 lime

- 2 tablespoons parsley, chopped

- 2 tablespoons pumpkin seeds

- 1 tablespoon basil, chopped

- 1 tablespoon balsamic vinegar

Directions:

1. In a slow cooker, combine the mushrooms with the tomatoes, olives, and the other ingredients, cook on low within 3 hours. Divide the salsa into bowls and serve as an appetizer.

Nutrition:

Calories: 129

Fat: 9.5g

Carbs: 9.4g

Protein: 5.4g

Onion Chickpeas Dip

Preparation time: 10 minutes

Cooking time: 2 hours

Servings: 4 people

Ingredients:

- 2 cups canned chickpeas, no-salt-added, drained and rinsed
- 1 cup red bell pepper, sliced
- 1 teaspoon onion powder
- 1 tablespoon lemon juice
- 1 teaspoon garlic powder
- 1 tablespoon olive oil
- 2 tablespoons white sesame seeds
- A pinch of cayenne pepper
- 1 and ¼ teaspoons cumin, ground

Directions:

1. In your slow cooker, mix red bell pepper with oil, sesame seeds, chickpeas, lemon juice, garlic and onion powder, cayenne pepper, cumin, cover, and cook on high for 2 hours. Transfer this mix to your blender, pulse well, divide into serving bowls and serve cold.

Nutrition:

Calories: 143

Fat: 3.8g

Carbs: 21.6g

Protein: 6.8g

Garlic and Beans Spread

Preparation time: 10 minutes

Cooking time: 6 hours

Servings: 4 people

Ingredients:

- 15 oz. canned white beans, no-salt-added, drained and rinsed
- 8 garlic cloves, roasted
- 1 cup low-sodium veggie stock
- 2 tablespoons lemon juice
- 2 tablespoons olive oil

Directions:

1. In your blender, mix beans with oil, stock, garlic, and lemon juice, cover the slow cooker, cook on low for 6 hours, transfer to your blender, pulse well, divide into bowls and serve as a snack.

Nutrition:

Calories: 214

Fat: 4g

Carbs: 33.2g

Protein: 12.9g

Sour Cream Dip

Preparation time: 20 minutes

Cooking time: 2 hours

Servings: 4 people

Ingredients:

- 1 bunch spinach leaves, roughly chopped

- ¾ cup low-fat sour cream

- 1 scallion, sliced

- 2 tablespoons mint leaves, chopped

- Black pepper to the taste

Directions:

1. In your slow cooker, mix the spinach with the scallion, mint, cream, and black pepper, cover, cook on high within 2 hours, stir well, divide into bowls and serve.

Nutrition: Calories: 121, Fat: 9.7g, Carbs: 6.3g, Protein: 4g

Simple Meatballs

Preparation time: 10 minutes

Cooking time: 8 hours

Servings: 16 meatballs

Ingredients:

- 1 and ½ pounds beef, ground

- 1 egg, whisked

- 16 oz. canned tomatoes, crushed

- 14 oz. canned tomato puree

- ¼ cup parsley, chopped

- 2 garlic cloves, minced

- 1 yellow onion, chopped

- Black pepper to the taste

Directions:

1. In a bowl, mix beef with egg, parsley, garlic, black pepper, and onion and stir well.

2. Shape 16 meatballs, place them in your slow cooker, add tomato puree and crushed tomatoes on top, cover, and cook on low within 8 hours. Arrange them on a platter and serve. Enjoy!

Nutrition:

Calories: 160

Fat: 5g

Carbs: 10g

Protein: 7g

Tasty Chicken Wings

Preparation time: 10 minutes

Cooking time: 3 hours

Servings: 6

Ingredients:

- 2 tablespoons garlic, minced
- 2 and ¼ cups pineapple juice
- 3 tablespoons coconut aminos
- 2 tablespoons tapioca flour
- 1 tablespoon ginger, minced
- 1 teaspoon sesame oil
- A pinch of sea salt
- 3 pounds of chicken wings
- A few red pepper flakes, crushed
- 2 tablespoons 5 spice powder
- Sesame seeds, toasted for serving

- Chopped cilantro, for serving

Directions:

1. Put 2 cups pineapple juice in your slow cooker, add sesame oil, a pinch of salt, coconut aminos, ginger, and garlic, and whisk well.

2. In a bowl, mix tapioca flour with the rest of the pineapple juice, whisk, and add to your slow cooker. Whisk everything and then add chicken wings.

3. Season them with pepper flakes and 5 spice, toss everything, cover and cook on high for 3 hours. Transfer chicken wings to a platter and sprinkle cilantro and sesame seeds on top.

4. Transfer sauce from the slow cooker to a pot and heat it for 2 minutes over medium-high heat. Whisk well, pour into small bowls, and serve your wings with it. Enjoy!

Nutrition: Calories: 200, Fat: 4g, Carbs: 9g, Protein: 20g

Chicken Spread

Preparation time: 10 minutes

Cooking time: 2 hours

Servings: 4 people

Ingredients:

- 12 oz. chicken breasts, skinless, boneless, cooked and shredded
- 10 oz. coconut cream
- 1 cup of coconut milk
- 1 cup hot sauce
- A pinch of salt and black pepper
- ½ teaspoon garlic powder
- ¼ cup scallions, chopped
- ½ teaspoon onion powder

Directions:

1. Mix the chicken with the cream, coconut milk, hot sauce, salt, pepper, garlic powder, scallions, and onion powder in your slow cooker, toss, cover, cook on low for 2 hours, stir again, divide into bowls and serve as a spread. Enjoy!

Nutrition:

Calories: 214

Fat: 4g

Carbs: 16g

Protein: 17g